USE THE WEIGHT TO LOSE THE WEIGHT

A REVOLUTIONARY NEW WAY TO LEVERAGE
THE STRENGTH YOU'VE DEVELOPED
CARRYING 50, 100, OR EVEN 150+ EXTRA
POUNDS AND CLAIM YOUR BAD-ASS STATUS
AS A REAL ATHLETE!

JOSH LAJAUNIE

HOWARD JACOBSON

INTRODUCTION: "WHEN I LOSE THE WEIGHT, THEN I'LL BE AN ATHLETE."

People often come up to me after hearing me talk, and they admire my story, but they can't actually relate to it. Instead, they feel like they can't self-identify as an athlete until they figure out how to go plant based and start moving and lose all of this weight. "When I'm healthy and thin, then I'll be an athlete."

And I get that, I understand that. I understand how society drives us to that way of thinking. But what I want people to understand and what I understand more now about my life and about what I've been through is that I *was* an athlete, not just at the first moment that I decided to step out into the gym and do something about losing all of this fat on my body.

I was an athlete all those years when I was morbidly obese.

I didn't realize it then, but I realize it now.

Yes, I might be a little slower than the other people at the gym, but they're not dealing with that same set of inputs that I was dealing with. There was no need for me to wait for a hundred pounds of weight loss to think of myself as an athlete at that point, because I was being more of a beast - more of an athlete - than anyone else in that gym.

Even at the very beginning of my weight loss journey, I was an athlete. I was lifting very heavy weights, in the form of my specific set of circumstances: physically, mentally, emotionally, familially (if that's a word), and societally for sure.

So a lot of people come up to me and they admire what I've done. They're inspired by me, but their narrative is, "Well, when I lose all this weight, then I'll start to be like Josh, then I'll start to be an athlete."

This book is about breaking that mindset apart, flipping it on its head and helping people move forward right now with a whole new mindset, with a whole new set of tools and protocols and practices.

You might be wondering: How does that mindset that people come in with - "Well, I'm fat now. I'm really out of shape. I'm not an athlete." – get in the way of progress? What's the big deal?

The big deal is it's hard to get up and be proud of your movement, be proud of what you're doing when you're constantly thinking you're not going to be able to consider yourself this powerful thing, this athlete, until you do your 100-pound weight loss worth of homework first.

That is very boring, that is very laborious. That is a heavy way to think about it.

But you can trick yourself (it's not really a trick because it's really the truth, but it feels like a trick because of societal pressures, because of the specific way we exist today).

You can trick yourself into understanding and believing the following:

"Hey, I am an athlete. I'm wearing a 200-pound weighted vest. If you threw that on the guy with the swole chest and ripped abs, he would struggle more than me because I am used to this. Therefore, I am a bigger beast of an athlete than he is - in my realm."

Rule your realm from day one and it'll help you tremendously and you will grow into that athletic persona that you're imagining right now without realizing what you already are.

Before you go out and start walking or running or lifting weights or doing yoga or anything, I want you to understand that what you're doing in your life right now is proportionally harder than some of the greatest athletic feats that we read about in the newspapers and see on TV.

To lose triple digit weight, to change your lifestyle, to take this body that's either chronically diseased or morbidly obese or both, and to put that physical machinery on the world's most elite athlete would bring him or her to his or her knees.

Yet you exist with that weighted vest on, every day of your life. You get on buses with it. You get on airplanes with it. You go to restaurants with booths with it and figure out how to get them to bring you a chair to the end of the table so you don't have to leave.

You exist with that in a way that this person who you are putting on a pedestal as some superior athlete could not even fathom.

They couldn't last two steps in your body.

So own that part of yourself, and let's slowly recommission it from mitigating this very heavy life. Let's recommission it to using its capacity for making us honestly, like an example for the people around us and something that we can be proud of inside of our own skin.

We don't have to wait into the future to be proud of ourselves.

Be proud of ourselves at step one, bite one and let's roll. Because even the beasts that you're looking at, myself included, couldn't handle that old weight vest of my old self if you threw it on me right now. I'm not adapted to that anymore. So in a crazy, weird, special, imaginative, creative way, you are a bigger beast than me.

I'm not even close. I've gotten soft.

Come get soft with me.

I want to highlight two really important points for you.

You're Not Lazy

First, even though the world might be telling you, overtly or subtly, "You're lazy. You have no self-discipline. You have no willpower. You're choosing the easy way out." - You're not.

The route you're taking now is harder than actually losing the weight and becoming an athlete. What you're doing now is more challenging than what "real athletes" do.

You're putting up with a lot of mental and emotional crap: the names, the talking behind the back, the hypersensitivity in your life and always thinking people are talking about you.

And you're also dealing with the physical drain of it: the physical weight of it every day. That's so much harder than the life I live now. I remember it. I've been both places.

You're in the Right Place Right Now

Second, where you are now is actually a really great place to start. It's almost like you're at the top of the mountain and you get to use gravity to bring you down easily, rather than having to climb the mountain.

Everything you think of as an obstacle is actually - when you look at it and use it in the right way - a tool that can help you become the kind of athlete you're thinking about more easily than someone who doesn't have all that weight.

Yes, you read that right. I thank my lucky stars for that 230-pound belly that I had to do something about.

I should say, that I had the *opportunity* to do something about it.

It – that big fat belly – is the thing that has grown me into a different man.

Into a better man.

In this book I'm going to take you on a little bit of a journey. In Chapter One I'm going to share my story. And not the *Runner's World* version of that story where I went from race to race, win to win, photo op to photo op, and smile to smile. Instead, I'm going to share the ugly parts, the disgusting parts, the micro of the ups and downs of that journey.

In Chapter Two I'm going to look at more specifically the challenges that come with starting to walk or run or work out. We'll explore why it's hard to move your body as a person with a lot of extra weight. You probably know all this, of course. So maybe this chapter is me trying to convince you that I understand what you're going through and what you're facing.

Then in Chapter Three I'm going to move on to solutions. And I'm going to start with mental solutions, with mindset. I'll show you how to change the way you think about certain things which will make everything you want a lot easier and a lot more approachable.

Chapter Four, I'll talk about what I call "flabby logistics": gear, clothing and other equipment that can make it easier for you to get moving with less discomfort.

Chapter Five, I'll look at the physical preparation your body needs before you start moving it with purpose and vigor. You'll learn about loosening up before working out, and about strengthening certain muscle groups that may have been underused for decades. Specifically, we'll be looking at opening the hips.

Chapter Six is all about the movement itself: specifically walking and running. You'll see how to get started, and how to not get ahead of yourself. We'll also explore specific aspects of form. If you've been overweight for a long time, you'll have to pay very close attention to form as you lose weight so you stop compensating for that big belly, for example.

In Chapter Seven, we'll look at how to recover after you've done your movement. How can you take care of your body so that it's capable of doing it again and again?

Chapters Four through Seven are pretty visual – tutorials on proper form, stretching, strengthening, and foam rolling, and demos of gear – so I've put together a video section at SicktoFit.com/usetheweight exclusively for readers of this book.

Chapters Eight and Nine are, in my mind, the heart of this book.

Chapter Eight is called "Fuck You." Vigorous, purposeful movement can actually be a "fuck you" to all the mean and negative voices in your head. The voices put there by other people: people who made fun of you when you were a kid; people who've doubted you; people who've put you down.

Because all those voices have taken up residence in your head, haven't they? Probably to the point that you think those voices are actually yours. You may think, like I did for many years, that you're the one telling you that you're just a fat ass.

That you're never going to do this. That you're too lazy. That you like sweets too much. While it's hard and often ineffective to try to argue rationally with those voices, movement can become an active "fuck you" to those voices and to those people.

Chapter Nine is the inverse of that. It's called "Love Me." I'll explain how that "fuck you" actually is a manifestation of great self-love. I'll show you how you can leverage that for your journey from fat to athlete.

Ready?

Let's jump in and get fit.

1

MY RUNNING BIO

I was 380 pounds the first time I decided to lace up and go outside and try this thing called running.

It felt so scary, so reckless and so irresponsible to put my big ass outside jogging on the ground. It seemed silly.

Nevertheless, I did it. I did it because I was being pragmatic and I thought it was going to help me and it did.

It was very difficult. It was hot during the summer. It made my shins hurt. It made my knees hurt, but it changed something in me. It made me more comfortable with discomfort.

It made me understand the value of the grind, of doing hard shit.

And of course, as I learned more and I got stronger and I got lighter, I started thinking of myself as an athlete. That was exhilarating to me.

I'd always been a fat guy who was on the line as a lineman playing football. That was my achievement, that was my goal. Get bigger so I could take on more offensive linemen or defensive linemen. And get in the way for the fit guys on the field.

When I started moving with the intent of getting faster, it was a very intoxicating elixir to feel light and fast; to feel that I could run like an animal.

And at the same time I realized, "Hey, I *am* a running animal. I'm a biped."

That's when I really bought in. I wanted that a lot.

I looked at other runners with "skins on the wall" that I wanted to be like. I did a lot of comparing early on, and I think it brought me to a sour place mentally without me realizing it.

I had just run my very organized road race in 2012. I had lost 50 or 60 pounds by that point. I had just graduated from college at the age of 29, and I really felt a sense of accomplishment. So I took my foot off the accelerator of progress. I kind of threw my heels up and relaxed a little bit, especially in the food department.

My weight started trending upward again, just like all the other times in my life after I'd made a concerted effort to drop pounds.

I was kind of aimless.

"What am I? Am I an ex-football player? Am I a businessperson who just graduated? Am I an employee now? Am I going to go get a job somewhere?"

I didn't know the answers. And from that place, I started questioning my new-found athletic identity.

"Am I a runner? Is that really what I am? Am I a healthy guy or am I just less fat? Is this what I'm meant to be?"

That was all of 2012. In 2013, my wife helped me choose and achieve a goal: "Let's run this race again, but let's do it a hell of a lot faster."

In that race, the 2013 Crescent City Classic 10k, there was a moment where I decided to let myself be irresponsible, to let myself feel reckless, to let myself go and run with the wind. It happened late in the race, when I was chasing her in pursuit of the goal of getting done in under an hour.

And that moment really changed me. I finished the race in 59 minutes and 57 seconds. We both achieved our sub-hour goal.

From there, my running really took off. I was hooked. In 2014, I did my first full marathon. My wife ran that with me. When 2015 rolled around, I ran my first ultramarathon, a 50k race (31 miles). That was awesome!

In mid-2016, I found myself thrown into this contest to get onto the cover of *Runner's World* magazine.

And yes, I had dealt with little nagging injuries along the way. The little rolled ankle, and the thing outside my knee hurts, and the IT band, and my low back is bothering me, but I had never been just completely debilitated.

By 2016 I was plant-based, and I felt like that was my bulletproof vest. I was really ignoring a lot of body things because I had my plant-based diet, and my body was going to recover. I knew it in my bones, so I let myself be reckless again, chasing something. And towards the end of 2016 right before the *Runner's World* photo shoot in my home town of Thibodaux, I hurt myself.

I really hurt my knee by ignoring all the pains during that time, because at that point I was trying to qualify for the Boston Marathon, and I was comparing myself to people whom I knew had already Boston qualified.

I was pushing myself hard, and I trying to prove that I'm pushing by sharing all of this information on the Internet, on the Strava app (a social media app for athletes), and I was doing all this to show everybody how much of an athlete I am.

What I know now is, it was elaborate mimicry that hurt me ultimately. While I was being praised on *Runner's World* for being some amazing story, I couldn't run the New York City Marathon that the cover reveal coincided with due to a swollen left knee, probably caused by a slightly torn meniscus. It was a bunch of swirling emotions, that was not good for me.

And then what came with winning the *Runner's World* cover contest was a free trip to Liverpool in May of 2017. So although I had to miss the New York City Marathon where all eyes were on me, I now had a chance to redeem myself in Liverpool, England on their dime.

Boy, that was enticing.

And so here I went again. As soon as I healed up enough to run at all with that knee, I was back out on the streets with this definite race coming up in May. And it didn't matter how bad I hurt, I needed a Boston qualifying time no matter what.

That's how it fits my plan. That's how it goes into my story:

"Josh is fat. He loses weight. He becomes a runner. He loses more weight. He runs a marathon. Then an ultra. He's on the cover of *Runner's World*. Not only has he done all this, but now he's Boston qualified."

How many people can say that they've done that?

So that was the focus, that was the goal.

That's what I was telling myself when I was hurting and pushing through the pain and being too tired to properly recover.

I was just too beat to foam roll or get massages or go to yoga or do any of the things that help with recovery. I just wanted that, that two letter hashtag: BQ.

The day came, and I didn't get it.

I didn't get it in Liverpool because all of those injuries - those little minor things that were really not minor at all - had compounded on me. They came to a head on race day.

Take an old football injury, aggravate it during the years of being heavy after football, add my new running passion, throw in six or eight months of running like a moron because I'm trying to ignore all of this physical pain.

The plan was, "I'm going to let it rest and recover. As soon as I get my BQ, then I'm going to chill."

And it didn't work out that way. Around mile 22 in the Liverpool Marathon I came completely apart. It wasn't my knee that bothered me. This time it was my back.

I twisted up. My whole body was wrenched because I'd been running kind of favoring one side.

Now, years later, I can talk about what happened because I've done a lot of homework in trying to figure out how I hurt myself. So I know now running like that kind of twisted my sacrum and then that hurt my lower back where I already had a bulging disc from football.

I can see clearly now, in hindsight, how this domino effect took place, from not caring for myself properly, for not thinking about myself the right way and not behaving the right way physically.

So what should have been a highlight of my life: my first trip to England, running a marathon, being feted as an amazing success on the cover of Runner's World. I spent the last four miles of that race walking a 15-minute pace, sobbing so hard that my abdomen was involved in a simultaneous muscle cramp.

The race was bad enough. I felt like I fell on my face in front of the whole world. I felt like I let down everybody who brought me to England via *Runner's World*.

It was debilitating. Not only that, but I allowed that experience to ruin what should have been an amazing trip to England with my lovely wife.

And when I got home, I stayed injured for months.

I couldn't run. I could hardly stand up straight. I couldn't sleep at night. It makes me want to cry just thinking about it. I went through months and months of sleepless nights and worrying, "Do I need surgery? Have I completely messed myself up?"

And in that process of me dealing with that at the same time, it became very abundantly clear that my grandfather, the man who essentially raised me, was going to die very soon. I could see it coming a couple months out. I could just feel it in my bones. So I went even deeper and darker towards the end of 2017 and sure enough, he died in August and I was still debilitated.

I couldn't run about it. I couldn't use movement to metabolize and express the pain I felt at his death. All I could do is just hurt and wonder when it's going to end.

I spent a lot of time Googling stuff, trying to find my own help because the traditional medical solutions for back pain fall short of anything fucking useful.

And to lump onto that, in December of that year, my damn beloved great Dane, Zeus, almost died on us and I had to spend enough money that I had to borrow money against my truck to fix him, to keep him from dying during Christmas.

And I say all of this not to make a sad sob story, but just to talk about the reawakening inside of me that has happened since then by turning a more self-loving eye to this thing I call life, which for me has become synonymous with running.

Zeus didn't die. That was a big step in the right direction emotionally for me. The clouds began to lift.

I began to understand more about myself as a runner. I discover that I like ultras more than marathons. Yes, I still want to Boston qualify. But I started to approach it with more self-compassion and love.

Here's how I began to explain it to myself: "Yeah, Josh, you haven't Boston qualified. Three hours and ten minutes is a very fast marathon. Yeah, Josh, those guys that you run with in Thibodaux, they're faster than you. They sure are. Both of them ran track in high school while you were knocking heads on the football field.

"Both of them kept up running recreationally after high school as a pastime while you went to the deer camp and drank half gallons of whiskey and ate steak and fried chicken and ate deer meat sand-wiches; while you was cutting up pigs; while you gained 230 pounds and lived a very toxic, poisonous life.

"So yeah, you didn't make it there yet, Josh, you haven't done that. True, but look at what you have done, son. Those motherfuckers can't touch it. They couldn't handle it."

I began to think about things more in that way. In early 2017, when I ran another ultramarathon with my friends, I was one of the last to finish the damn thing. It took me eight hours and 30 minutes, but I wanted to be an ultrarunner again. I wanted to make sure I was still that and I was.

Boston will always be there and I'll always keep it as a North star, but I'm not going to let it toxify how I think about myself and how much I've achieved. It took walking through some ugly places in my life and some dark nights to turn that tide inside. Getting a new coach, taking a new approach on my runs, switching up running partners.

All of these things changed as my self-love and self-awareness and self-compassion sort of really came into focus. Even though I had lost all of this weight and achieved all of these "athletic things," I was still broken because I don't think I was really thinking of myself just right yet.

I have taken a different approach in my running since those days. I have pulled back the intensity, I only do one sort of intense workout a week now. I have slowed way down on many of the other workouts. I spend a lot more time helping myself recover, hugging myself, loving myself with the foam roller or with added strength, with pull-ups and pushups and just different strength things I can do in the gym instead of constantly feeling like the tachometer has to be at 8000 RPMs so I can catch those fast guys to prove that a fat guy can do that.

Fuck, I've proved shit that a fat guy already thinks is impossible. I have to understand that now and turning that eye inward, turning that loving eye inward, that aspirational eye inward.

I've purposely put blinders on, to stop comparing myself to the people that I've been comparing myself to, even my very closest buddies. That has helped me grow in a new way in the past year or so of my life.

And lo and behold, my running strength is getting back. I'm becoming just as fast as I was before I hurt myself. Now I feel like I've actually got a real fire burning. It's not just a grease fire. We've got some good deep organic charcoal that burns a long time.

And it all is just a perpetual evolution: a bubbling and mixing of feelings and thoughts and purposeful action that are all oriented towards better, towards growing.

Sometimes what we think of as better, as growth, actually can be towards a toxic place. It was for me; I had to bump against it and learn about it, take a turn and move into a healthier direction.

But at the core of it all, we have to start with that first inkling of self-respect. And that happened for me very early on in that moment with my wife, in that very first Crescent City Classic and that very first race. And so although I have been through tons of toxic situations inside my own self and externally as well, I am eternally thankful for the lessons in that very first race I ever did. Not only that, I'm grateful for all of the mistakes that I have made along the way, since then that I'm able to talk to you about right now.

And although I'm older, I'm probably going to start getting slower, maybe not a whole lot more podium finishes in my future, I have to say I love myself and the athlete that I am and I respect him more than I ever have in my life. Whether I was faster or slower, fatter or thinner.

And that has got to be one of the best feelings a person can have. And without running, and the difficulty and mistakes and hurt associated with it, I really honestly don't think I would be here.

So understand that getting started moving, especially as a heavy person, it's not gumdrops and lollipops and rainbows and unicorns and fuzzy things to hug.

There's shit.

And not only is it okay, but that shit will fertilize your growth if you love it, if you turn your attention towards it, if you're present for solutions that show their head along the way.

So embrace the difficulty of growth and learn that your self-love is an evolutionary process. As you get up, improve it day after day.

I don't know how else to better get out of me what is inside of me other than to do what I'm doing right now: to talk to you about it. And I hope inside my heart of hearts that it resonates in some small way with someone and helps me plant a seed.

You bring the shit.

2

WHAT THEY DON'T TELL YOU ABOUT GETTING FIT WHEN YOU'RE FAT

So yeah, I was heavy. I've been heavy all my life.

If you're also heavy, then you've heard the stories about how you should lose weight, about how you should get healthy. You hear those sentiments from others, mostly in innuendo, but sometimes in your face.

Does this one sound familiar?: "I don't care about how big you are, I just care about your health."

And you're probably hosting all those conversations all by yourself, in your own head, all the time.

And every so often you take action, and you lose weight – for a while. You try really hard, disciplining and depriving yourself, going on diets and off diets, going down and up in weight.

It's very frustrating. Over time, highest weight gets heavier and heavier, until you finally start to do something about it for real. You finally start losing weight in a sustainable way.

I say "you," but of course I mean "me." I just told you my story. Yours may be similar.

And what no one ever tells you – certainly what no one ever told me - is that being fat is basically an extreme sport.

And losing that fat is even more extreme.

Being Fat is an Extreme Sport

I was 230 pounds overweight. That weight was bearing me down and mashing me to the earth.

It was hurting – and damaging - the pressure points on my knees and ankles.

And with that much extra flesh, just moving my body in space took a huge toll. Fat people have to use their limbs in a different way than normal folks. I had so much fat between my thighs that my bones hung from my hips in a different way than most people.

When my right leg wanted to swing, I couldn't just pick it up and bring it forward. Instead, it had to first swing around the fat on the left leg and on the right leg. There were two big globs of fat that my bones had to swing around for me to walk, which torqued the hips and the lower back in all sorts of different ways that your skinny friends don't have to deal with.

If you and a skinny friend start a walking program tomorrow, they'll have it much easier than you. You'll both by moving and sweating, but they may seem to be progressing at a faster rate. That's because they're not dealing with these giant obstacles.

Being obese for a long time doesn't affect just the musculo-skeletal system. I've struggled with recovering recently, so I had some blood tests done and discovered that my liver was genetically compromised.

Turns out I was born with a not particularly rare condition called Gilbert's syndrome. And that discovery led me to find out more about what the liver actually does. I started to realize how I've taxed my liver over the years.

I catalogued all the poison I had subjected it to: the high fat meals, the whiskey, the recreational drugs, the pharmaceutical drugs taken either recreationally to get high, or taken because the doctor told me to take it because my back's hurting too bad or because I'm sick or because I'm not feeling good. The drugs I used to take for depression. And the anxiety and stress and constant adrenaline generated by my thinking back in those days.

Getting Thin is Even More Extreme

Once I started moving in the direction of health and a right-sized body, I discovered that process is also taxing and toxifying and demanding. That turned out to be really tricky mentally.

"Hey, I'm doing all the right things; why is my body hurting so much? Why am I more fatigued and achy and distracted now than it was when I was abusing it with my diet and lifestyle?"

Coming back to my liver – I would have thought that improving my diet, laying off the drugs and alcohol, and reducing my weight would be great for liver function.

Not to mention all the extra stuff that I did, that I wanted to pat myself on the back for doing. Losing 230 pounds. Becoming a runner, then a marathoner, now an ultramarathoner.

I should be healthy now, dammit!

But here I am, and my liver enzymes are still high. Sure, I've got this Gilbert's Syndrome, which is going to manifest elevated liver enzymes. But beyond that, my liver was also taxed by the effort of metabolizing all the crap that I had been ingesting for decades.

The liver, I discovered, deals with a toxic load in the body by storing as much of the poison as it can in fat cells.

When I started losing that weight, my liver had to deal with those toxins all over again. They'd been neutralized by being stored in fat; now they were back in my bloodstream, wreaking havoc, requiring my poor, genetically compromised, brutally abused liver to work overtime to keep me alive.

When I told Howie about my liver issues and my research, he said something that really resonated with me on a deep level: "The poison stings on the way in and it stings on the way out."

That was a very powerful concept for me. It helped me see that my fatigue and pain wasn't a weird anomaly. I was thinking, "I've done all this and now what? I still have a problem." I had been kind of bitter about it, to be honest. Like it was unfair and inexplicable.

Now I had a better narrative.

My liver, which was born compromised and which I had abused for 32 years, had a lot of heroic work to do *because* I had created the conditions under which the toxins could finally leave me body.

Realistically, it took me 32 years to put that amount of poison into my body. The fact that I've reversed so much of that damage in six or eight is pretty bad ass. I'm on a really good trajectory. And yes, I understand that my poison hurt as it comes out a little bit more. I understand that, but that means to me also that it's temporary. It's solvable.

So take that process seriously, and be in awe of your body a little bit as it compensates and heals and finds workarounds for all the physiological systems that you've damaged along the way. You're taxing your body at least as much when you're getting *un*fat as you did when you were getting fat in the first place.

But there's more. You're still going to experience those physical and environmental challenges that all fat people face long after you've started losing weight.

If you were 200 pounds overweight, and you lost 100 of those pounds, that's amazing! You should feel justifiably proud of yourself.

And...

You still have 100 excess pounds that are weighing you down and compromising your joints. Pounds that are still messing with your center of gravity and throwing off your gait.

It's still hard to go up and down stairs. It's hard to get comfortable on a bus, or in a booth seat in a restaurant, or on an airplane, or in a theater.

Yes, you're doing great, and you're still overweight, with all the problems and challenges that go along with excess poundage. That's a very weird place to live. It's very frustrating. Be gentle with yourself at this point on your journey.

And at the same time, DO NOT get complacent. Look your ongoing challenge in the eye.

"Yes, I've lost a hundred pounds, but I am not done yet, and that's okay."

It's okay that it feels burdensome. Instead of resenting that burden, I want you to start appreciating all of these things, the challenges, the hard parts, the difficult parts, the things that don't seem damn fair.

This is how you stop making yourself feel bad and inadequate when you compare yourself to others.

Take a moment to appreciate all of the shit you're dealing with that other people aren't. Stop beating yourself up for doing a 16-minute mile on a treadmill right now. Stop beating yourself up for being tired when you "only" walked three miles yesterday. Understand that your three miles is a much bigger deal than your skinny neighbor's three miles.

Yes, you all both started last week. So what? Time is not the only input.

When you understand how hard your body has been working all these years, and how hard it's working now that you're turning the ship around, you can finally appreciate these challenges as not only OK, but vital to your growth and success.

Turning a loving eye towards these very ugly, toxic, poisonous parts of the journey will free your heart and soul and allow you to finally embrace that self that's going to, not drag you out of this, but very lovingly and pragmatically lead you out of this stuck place you may have found yourself.

That's the mindset that empowers you to take a next step forward; a step from which there's no going back.

3

YOUR MENTAL GAME

I f you're on social media, you've probably seen a bunch of accounts that are all about self-love.

Mostly, these folks talk about loving yourself the way you are, and I think that's beautiful. I really do.

Beware of Pseudo Self-Love

But I think the way people interpret and operationalize that sentiment, it gets lost in the woods of something not so useful. We can twist the idea of self-love into an excuse not to better ourselves.

As in, "I love myself exactly as I am, so there's no need to change."

As in, any talk of obesity being unhealthy becomes a toxic form of "fat-shaming."

That kind of pseudo self-love talk just keeps us stuck, and in truth, miserable.

If you loved a baby, you'd feed her healthy food. You'd change her dirty diapers. You wouldn't give her beer and chicken nuggets and let her lay there in day-old shit and piss and explain, "But I love her just the way she is."

That's not love.

And when you look at how you've treated yourself over the years, all the indulgences and poor choices and compulsions and addictions and whatever, you see clearly that isn't self-love.

And continuing to do those things, even under the guise of a new rhetoric of "body positivity," isn't self-love either.

Self-love isn't a word, it's a protocol.

It's an ongoing set of decisions and actions in which you treat yourself like someone in your care.

True Self-Love

True self-love starts with a total surrender to reality; an acceptance that where you are right now is OK. And that you're OK for being here, right now.

Meaning, you don't have to beat yourself up or shame yourself or criticize yourself or yell at yourself to make progress. And you don't have to pretend that you aren't where you're at.

If you're too fat to get off the sofa, if you can't fit in a booth at a restaurant, if putting on socks feels like a cardio workout - wherever you are, that's where you must start.

And not just start there and begrudgingly accept it or surrender to it. Because begrudging acceptance is really resistance with a pretty bow around it. "Yeah, I'm here, but I wish I wasn't. I don't like being here, but I guess pragmatically I have to tolerate it for the time being."

No.

I'm talking about starting where you are and actually for the first time in your fucking life, love it, embrace it, appreciate it. Finally, see the assets and all the good things that you are, instead of only the liabilities and the ugly pieces.

Finally, being able to understand that, yes, I have slipped this far, but I can get off the elevator right now. There's no need to go all the way to the bottom.

The Power in the Decision

That moment when you decide to change is huge.

When you make that "athletic decision" to start moving, and to start moving forward, that's not a fat person trying to be fit.

That's a fit person trying to get out.

Understand that, love that. Appreciate that fit person, and shake your head in awe of the work that fit person is willing to do to unpeel that fat suit and get healthy.

Reject Comparisons

True self-love doesn't compare you to anyone else.

Don't let comparison rob you of the joy that changing brings. Start exactly where you are and embrace the capacity that you currently possess.

Don't denigrate that capacity, or dismiss the mountain that you have just set out to climb, by comparing yourself to others. Comparisons are excruciating, especially in the beginning of your journey to fitness, whether you're comparing yourself to athletes who have been on this journey longer than you, or to other people losing weight.

Aside from being discouraging and demoralizing, there's a pragmatic reason to reject the comparisons that your mind wants to make to put you down and weaken your resolve: they're completely wrong.

You simply don't have enough data to make a fair comparison with anyone else.

There is no way for you to know everyone else's different sets of inputs. You'll always be comparing apples to oranges.

How do you know what it feels like for someone else to run a 12-minute mile?

How do you know if someone else's liver is more efficient at metabolizing fat than yours is?

How do you know if someone else gets much deeper sleep than you do?

You simply can't make educated, accurate comparisons. So stop doing it, because you're wrong. You're making huge-ass assumptions with no evidence to back them up.

If you think about it, you're making these bullshit comparisons for one reason only: to get out of doing the work.

You may not realize it at the time, but consider where the thought cascade ends when you start by comparing yourself to someone else who's "doing better" than you are. You end up demoralized.

And that's the prelude to self-pity.

And self-pity is the fuel for all your bad habits, all the self-hating self-indulgences that got you to this point.

So reject the mental habit of comparison, which Teddy Roosevelt called "the thief of joy," and instead choose self-love.

Comprehensive self-love, that includes embracing who you are and where you are right now.

Love the One You're With

You're going to love that person because that's the person who's going to get you through. That's the person who's going to do all the hard, unpleasant, unsexy work that's going to give you the life you want.

And five years from now, you're going to look back and say, "Josh was right. I love that person so much. Thank you so much for dancing with me, person. Thank you so much for taking that first step. Thanks for getting those bloody nipples on your first runs. Thank you so much for being willing to hurt for me. Thank you for ignoring all of the naysayers and telling them, 'Fuck you.'"

Ultimately, losing weight is a mental game. The mechanics are simple. Change the inputs in terms of food and physical activity. If you want guidance on those fronts, check out our first book, *Sick to Fit*.

Doing those things consistently is mental.

Being happy is mental.

That's easy enough to say. But it begs the question, how do you hone your mental game? There's no magic button to press to give yourself a positive mindset. There's no anti-depressant that actually makes you happy.

The best way to hone your mental game is to keep making those decisions to love yourself. To consistently take those actions that manifest that love.

You can't always (or perhaps ever) control your thoughts. But you can often control your actions.

Let's say you have this thought, "I'm a fat piece of shit." And no amount of therapy is helping to dismantle or defang that thought. And you read this chapter about mindset and now you feel even worse about having that thought. What to do?

Start acting like someone who believes, "I'm a human being, worthy of love and care."

Feed yourself healthy food.

Move your body with purpose, every day.

So even while your mind is going, "I'm a piece of shit, I'm a piece of shit," your eyes are seeing evidence to the contrary. Your actions are undermining your shitty narrative, day in and day out.

That's the true gym for the mind. Not affirmations and memes and motivational posters. But actions that align with self-love.

Actions that prove self-love.

Actions that *are* self-love.

Making those decisions to love yourself and be happy and find joy in life, there's no better way to hone your mental game. Because while mindset without action is meaningless, action that doesn't change mindset is unsustainable.

If you think that you can change your life and find all this happiness with physical inputs only, you're going to have a rude awakening. You've probably already had that awakening many times in your life. The diet, the gym routine – they didn't last because you didn't use them in an intentional way to upgrade your mindset.

You were throwing away most of their power.

So I invite you to embrace the difficult parts of honing your mental game. Embrace yourself for where you are, as difficult as that may be right now.

Lock hands with that person, and walk with them, step for step, into the future together. It sounds silly, but that's how I roll. it's not just my voice in my head. I have a team that's on my side in my head battling those old voices that say I can't.

As you'll see in Chapter 8, those old voices that put me down are really just ideas I've accidentally adopted from assholes in my life. I combat those negative voices by inviting, in a deliberate and purposeful way, positive voices that can gang up on the assholes and drown them out.

Thinking by Moving

Inside of this big joyful dance that I'm talking about is another smaller dance. It's the dance of finally listening to your physical body.

If you're like me, you have been living in your head for a very long time.

And so it's a very nuanced thing to learn your body: to feel it, to understand swelling and bruising and little nagging aches, and pains and sore muscles and tight areas. These may all seem like trivial issues, or maybe not so trivial depending on how bad you hurt, but in any case tangential to the big picture.

But they're not trivial or tangential. Instead, these ordinary physical sensations are the brushstrokes that make up the big picture.

You've been trying to envision the Mona Lisa, this perfect future version of yourself, in concept only.

Now it's time to open the paint tubes and start getting messy.

Now it's time to deal with body sensations through physical move-ment. Whatever the issue is, the answer is not to lay on the sofa until that thing goes away.

The answer is to just downgrade your intensity to a level that allows you to heal through whatever it is you're dealing with at the moment.

That requires a nuanced understanding of your body. And that only grows with experience.

I like to compare that process to a dance, because you are dancing with your body to create new outcomes. Dancing yourself in a new direction.

And only you and your body can hear that music. To someone on the outside looking in, they may think that you're dancing all dumb looking, but in reality you're the only one that can really hear and feel the beat.

So dance the weight away. Pay attention to your body and ignore the naysayers.

4

THE LOGISTICS OF BEING FLABBY

I didn't realize that losing weight would make me flabby.

I thought that I was doing great – and I was. I had lost 150 pounds, the most I'd ever lost in my life.

And strangely, that was when my body image was at its worst. I was "maximum flab" at that point.

Because before, the flab had sort of been "fleshed out" with fat. Now it was just hanging lose everywhere, flapping and flopping whenever I tried to move.

Of course, there was plenty of flab in the early days of my movement journey, when I weighed close to 400 pounds.

When I started walking and "jiggle jogging," I discovered that my extra weight was problematic not just in terms of the "carry me around all day" effect. It did all sorts of annoying things when in motion.

And as a pragmatic Coonass (what some of us Cajuns from the bayou call ourselves as a term of endearment), I discovered and invented tricks to keep that flab from making my life too miserable, starting with the very first Crescent City Classic I ran in 2012, at over 300 pounds.

Flab in Motion

When you start moving while fat, you'll discover a whole world of sound and kinetics that happens. There's jigging and clapping and slapping and flopping. There's painful chafing that occurs when parts rub against each other while "lubricated" by sweat.

Those unpleasantries, those minor "benign" injuries, helped teach me how to navigate this part of the journey and make them a lot less annoying and painful. So in this chapter I'm going to share what I've learned with you.

Maybe it will spare you a few bloody nipples. If so, that's cool. But my real intention here is to keep you on the path, to smooth out what I can so you continue moving forward, making progress, growing stronger and faster and more athletic.

The Magic of Compression

Here's a Fat Boy trick my brother and I used to pull at fancy events like weddings and funerals to appear slightly less fat. We would buy a plain white t-shirt one size too small, and wear it under our suit.

When I ran my very first race, I borrowed that trick to keep my belly in place. I took that too-small and cut off the sleeves. When I tucked that undershirt into my pants and put on a regular t-shirt, you couldn't tell that I was wearing it.

Think of it as an early version of "Spanx for men." Dustin, we could have been billionaires!

Except it wasn't some fancy and expensive compression garment; it was a Hanes cotton T- shirt that was just too small for me. I used it as a sausage case on my big body so I wouldn't be clapping and flapping as I ran past people or they ran past me.

That was my first lesson in the usefulness of compression, especially as a fat person on their way to being fit and thinner and leaner and having less need for these things.

I say "less" because you will probably need compression for the rest of your running existence, even after you lose triple digit weight.

For example, as I got further along in my running and lost even more weight, I started to develop chafing at the lower ass cheek area and inner thigh. My thighs would literally just rub the skin off one another because I was wearing traditional running shorts with just the netting in them.

I started experimenting. I tried wearing longer boxer briefs instead of just regular tidy whities (what we would call on the bayou "coson").

Actual Compression Gear

Then I discovered actual compression gear for runners, and tried just about every brand and style out there. Skinny runners use them to regulate blood flow in various parts of their bodies, but for fat people, they serve another purpose.

You may not even realize you want to know this, but compression shorts are a wonderful tool to keep your thighs tucked in and to keep your ass cheeks pressed together so they don't flop and rub when you get really sweaty and create the chafing that happens there.

One piece of advice: most of us buy compression pants that are too small for us. We don't need to lock it all down and immobilize our mid-sections. All we want is to restrict the movement of skin and flesh that will lead to chafing.

Another issue with compression pants is that most of them have waistbands that are too skinny for us fat and formerly fat people. A skinny waistband will just dig into your soft ooey-gooey midsection. As your run progresses, it keeps digging and digging, and it sort of rolls itself up and forms a cord around your belly and is zero fun to deal with.

The wider the waistband, the better.

And what I have found as the best pair, because it hits all the good attributes for me is a brand called Shock Doctor, the manufacturer of athletic cups. But those athletic cups come with this compression short that has a really wide nice waistband that rests softly against your skin, and doesn't dig in.

It may take a couple of purchases to find your right size. But I would recommend finding the longest pair you can find that stays above the knee, compression shorts with the widest waistband you can find. Heck, even maternity clothes will work.

The most important thing is to quiet down the wiggly jigglyness. Not just to avoid skin abrasion or trauma when you're starting out, walking slowly, but also as you get to work and move forward.

After a while, what was impossibly hard becomes pretty easy and unchallenging. At that point, you'll want to ramp up your effort so you keep making progress. As you "outgrow" slow walking and aspire to go faster, or longer, or both, it becomes even more important to keep the jiggles at bay.

The more active and aggressive you get, the more dynamically your flab will swing. And even though there's a lot less of it than when you started, it's still soft and wiggly jiggly.

The more you want to speed up, the more all that lateral and up-and-down swinging of flesh and fat and flab will interfere with your forward motion. Compression clothing will calm that all down and keep your mass moving as a unit, always forward.

You may also find compression shirts useful for keeping belly and boobs from swinging. I've never tried Spanx for me, but 2XU brand makes compression shirts that will be better than a tight cotton tee-shirt, especially if you'll be sweating a lot. Cotton retains water, and wet cotton can be really uncomfortable when you run for a long time.

In 2014, I ran the New York City Marathon with a 2XU compression shirt under my singlet.

Compression of the upper body not only helps you quiet down some of the physical skin trauma, but it can also help you just feel more together and feel more okay with people seeing you as you walk, jog, or run.

I believe that in a perfect world it wouldn't matter what others think, but it kind of does a little bit. I understand and I'm giving truth to that dynamic. I know that you care about that.

There's one more area of compression that I would like to talk about: the arms. This was a big thing for me. In the beginning, my arms were still so fat that I was worried about wearing sleeveless stuff.

But if you're running or jogging a 10K in the middle of summertime, you don't want to wear long sleeves. You don't want to close off your arm pits. It would be nice to wear a muscle shirt, but if your upper arm has gotten so fat that it has its own belly, and its own set of loose skin that hangs down around the elbow, you will want to do something about that.

Running stores often sell arm sleeves, which are exactly what they sound like: long sleeves that you can put on and take off independent of a shirt. You may like those, but they may not be necessary. Here's another place where you can get creative, and experiment.

If you already own compression socks or calf sleeves (which are more for keeping the blood flowing than preventing jiggling), try those on your arms. Cut the sleeves off an old Under Armor shirt.

Why experiment?

Because you are doing something in rarified air. There haven't been many who have come before us in this journey. The world is not prepared for us. There aren't a lot of companies making athletic clothing and gear for folks our size. We have to make our own way sometimes, and it's okay. It's all right.

You're going to relish these efforts later on, especially when you can share them with other folks. It's a beautiful full circle moment. The main thing is, don't beat yourself up for still being flabby. Expect it, accommodate it, and experiment to mitigate it. And share what works with those who follow you, just like I'm doing.

People are understandably fascinated with my stretch marks, especially after they see a really dramatic before-and-after photo montage. They think of skin as a static thing, like a shirt. They imagine my skin as a 5XLT shirt now draped like a tablecloth over this lean L body.

Here's what they don't really understand: your skin is dynamic. It is alive.

That means you're not flabby permanently. As you lose weight, your skin has less fat to hold, so it's in a transition phase between being puffed out and swollen with fat and being lean with a little bit of extra skin and some stretch marks.

But between being so fat that you're at risk of dying any day of a heart attack and being lean with just extra skin and stretch marks, there is a considerable period of time where you will be flabby. And that's perfectly normal, and it's OK.

Don't be tempted to cut that extra skin off. I've seen it too many times.

Your skin will shrink as you continue to burn away fat. You'll be surprised.

Use compression, be prepared for that awkward flabby transition time, and keep moving your body to keep mobilizing and metabolizing body fat.

We're being pragmatic about this. We see a problem, we're solving it. We don't need a special "fat person gear store."

No need to feel sorry for ourselves: "Boy, if they just had a place where we could get all this stuff."

No, we are creating it for ourselves. Be part of this crowdsourced experiment with me. I'm doing the best I can to help you and show you what to do specifically when you're dealing with this transitional phase. Don't shy from it. Understand that flabby is okay, and we can creatively and pragmatically deal with it to continually make ourselves stronger physically and emotionally.

Other Anti-Flabby Supplies

Compression can help with chafing, as we've seen, but there are other things you can use as well. Compression doesn't really help with the bloody nipples that are so common when you really ramp up the time and distance of your runs, especially when it's hot out.

I have so much extra skin on my chest that it slides up and down, and rubs against the inside of my shirt. If I go more than four or five miles, my nipples get really tender and start to bleed.

I tried multiple things, but what I found worked for me the best is Scotch tape. A little perfectly square piece of opaque Scotch tape right on my nipple and boom, problem solved. That may work for you, and it may not work. Experiment and see. You might prefer a different kind of tape, or a Band Aid, or a lubricant like Body Glide or petroleum jelly.

Pay attention to where you get little rashes after your runs. Those are your chafing hot spots. Smear some Body Glide or Vaseline on them before your next run.

If you get blisters on your toes, find a product called Trail Toes and rub it all over your toes before you put your socks on so you don't create any friction and blisters.

No matter what your particular issue or discomfort, there are ways around this. We're going to get through this flabby phase, and we're going to get to the other side of it.

And we're going to be fit, lean, running together, changing the world. Don't let your belly clapping at you get you down. As we've seen, there are plenty of ways around it.

And understand that it's really just your body giving you a round of applause.

5

PHYSICAL PREPARATION FOR MOVEMENT

I t's great to get started on this journey. We can move our body in aggressive ways, and we can tease it into shedding body fat. We can overcome soreness, we can have a better mindset around what we're doing. We can mitigate and recover from all the little nagging pains that come along.

But it's also very important to prepare, to warm your body up before moving. I don't just hop out of my truck and go for a run. Whatever your workout is, don't just jump right into it. Take it slow. Loosen yourself up. Love yourself into this movement – think of it like foreplay for your body.

I've already explained how your biomechanical structure gets deviated from its natural "normal" because of all of this extra body fat. It's very important to prepare for jogging or running by deliberately moving your hips in a way that they're not used to move.

Your hips don't want to do that because when you're heavy, your hips require stability far more than mobility. They "think" they need to be still. So you lock up your sacrum and your sacroiliac (SI) joints, along with your entire your lumbar spine, and you get very stiff there. That's natural, and probably a useful adaptation if you're really heavy.

But once you start moving, and you start losing weight, it's really important to slowly and carefully begin to mobilize that area, and all the joints in it. If not, if you start moving more vigorously and you keep that middle part really stiff, you can pretty much tear yourself apart.

What happens is, your low back and hips are supposed to move as you run. If they are locked up, other parts of your body have to over-compensate, which can cause pain and damage in areas far away from where the problem is. It's not uncommon for my chiropractor to deal with ankle, knee, or shoulder pain by mobilizing my right hip, for example.

Tight hips and back have been a big contributor to the pain and injuries I've dealt with over the past couple of years.

I'm finally understanding how tight I let my hips get. The best way I've found for increasing my hip mobility has been good, deep static squats.

Picture a human in their indigenous environment, maybe Papua New Guinea or somewhere in Africa. Can you see them sitting in a squat, their feet flat on the ground, with their hips and torso basically hanging from their knees? That's a very natural human posture. It's simple, and far more authentic than sitting on an office chair, couch, or recliner.

It's a key piece of our evolutionary heritage, and the fact that I can't get anywhere close to that posture speaks volumes to me about my unnatural life up to this point.

Like me, you probably won't be able to sit in a full squat right now. Your best option is to do an assisted squat, maybe holding the back of a chair, or a doorknob, or pulling on a resistance band attached to a door or wall.

Get into as deep a squat as feels safe, and hang out (literally) for as long as you can. At first, it might just be a few seconds. See if you can turn that into minutes through repetition. Keep breathing into the tightest spots, and on the exhales, see if your body will allow you to go slightly deeper into the stretch.

Never force it. Remember, it's foreplay, not assault.

I understand now how being heavy, and then being a heavy runner, and then being an ultra runner has seized up and locked my hips and low back in a lot of ways.

As I heal up from my 2017 injury, I've discovered that loosening my body up before I get started moving is critical.

Free Your Body Up Before Movement

Slowly warm your body up, even if it's just a little bit of walking to start. Then maybe move to a little bit of toe hopping. Figure out your own protocol to address your own chronically tight, stuck, and immobilized areas, but don't skip it because you want to get your "real" movement in and you're in a rush.

Move your body through different planes. Up and down; side to side; twisting upper and lower body in different directions. Really focus on opening up those hips. And every chance you get, go into one of those deep assisted squats where you hang out and try to mimic the people in National Geographic magazine for a minute or two.

Strength Training

Another area to focus on to help your body get prepared to move with aggression is strength.

You may think that your muscles are really strong because of all those years you went around wearing a triple-digit fat suit, and some of them are, but others – really important muscles – are weak to the point of atrophy. I guarantee it.

For example, I discovered that my ass has really atrophied and gotten very weak because I was using other muscles to balance out my giant belly.

After talking to numerous running coaches and physical therapists and trainers and chiropractors and massage therapists, I started noticing that most of my running issues could be traced to weak gluteus maximus muscles.

My stride problems? Weak ass.

My heel pain? Weak ass.

Back pain? You get the idea.

It took me a while, but I finally understood the power of that muscle. The gluteus maximum, the big muscle in our ass, is our running muscle, our climbing muscle. It's crucial to get it firing.

And so not only do we want to strengthen it with weights and running and stair climbing, but we want to make sure that we use the strength that we already have in there by turning that muscle on with the brain.

So spend time on YouTube, learning about how to activate and strengthen the gluteus maximus.

Find a trainer or a physical therapist or body worker who can help you help you identify what muscles are not only weak, but also those that may be strong but are just turned off.

You probably have muscles that just aren't firing because you haven't used them for years, maybe because like me you've been getting yourself up out of chairs like a pregnant lady because of your big belly.

My nerd friend Howie tells me that the fancy term for this is "Sensory

Motor Amnesia." It's like your brain has just forgotten about those muscles, which are nevertheless in perfect shape and raring to go.

So as you're loosening joints and to increase mobility, you also want to get stronger and stronger to give yourself a favorable "strength to weight" ratio. In other words, the stronger your muscles, the lighter your body is proportionate to your strength. That's a shortcut to upgrading your physical machinery, making yourself fitter and fitter and raising your capacity in a virtous cycle.

Growing Your Strength

I love the idea of running because it seems like such an innate natural human movement. That said, in addition to the focusing on gaining flexibility in the hips and back and legs, and increasing cardiovascular capacity by running faster and and farther, gaining just sheer power is important as well. Especially, I have found, in my upper back and chest area.

I love the idea of being able to lift my own body weight. That would look like a lot of things: getting myself up out of a chair without using my arms, or doing my first pushup on my toes instead of my knees, or being able to hang from a pullup bar for 30 seconds for the first time.

Developing a growth mindset about the strength of your whole body is just as important as what we eat and how far you walk or run or jog. You have turned muscles off that you need to turn back on. You've misused muscles because of those two big fat pillows between your thighs, and the muscles on the outside of your hip sockets probably work in a way that they're not used to because they've been swinging around.

You have muscles that have atrophied and have muscles that have been overworked. Here's what I've discovered: building whole body strength goes beyond hitting all the planes of motion and loosening the hips and all the physical protocols I'm sharing with you here.

Really building whole body strength goes hand in glove with the self love we were talking about in Chapter 3. This is how we set the table for the growth necessary to become what we dream.

The more strength we have, the more capacity we have to not only help us move this body around the earth, but to help be of use to those around us.

Just a small example: I went to a farm animal sanctuary rescue this weekend and it felt amazing. It's not like I've been working out for five years to go haul logs for these people on this farm, but it felt amazing to take all of the physical capacity that I've built to lose 230 pounds, run ultra marathons, get myself on the cover of Runner's World, and all of these selfish things, and use it to do some hard labor for animals.

It would have felt just as good if I had gone and helped at an old folks home or at an orphanage. Remember that you're building strength and capacity and mobility not just for yourself. Think about some way you could volunteer or help out or contribute to some individual or group or cause that you care about, but that you can't do right now. Think about how good it will feel to deploy your new-found capacity in that kind of service.

Don't let yourself stop at thinking of movement as just a way to make your stronger so your exercise and your running can be better. Understand that loving yourself through these physical things to move you forward is exactly what you need to do to help change the world. That's the way I look at it anyway. So stay focused, and stay pragmatic.

Stay in a position of love, and not just for yourself. When you think about yourself moving through this process, don't shy away from or feel selfish about wanting to be strong and powerful.

That strength and powerful will be not just be used by you. Other people around you, other beings around you, will be better off for you having gotten more physically prepared for movement.

It's Not a Contest

As an ex-football player who used to measure myself by what I could bench press or dead lift, I want to emphasize that strength training is not a contest. Neither is stretching or loosening.

Whether you're doing it on your own, or going to a yoga class, or working out at the gym, you're not trying to set new records or beat anyone else. The contest has shifted; now it's life itself.

Having a healthy, vibrant, service-based, loving, happy life. That's the contest, not who can do yoga better or who can get into a deeper squat. We want to love ourselves through these movements because they are going to propel us forward through the physical movement.

And authentic, within-our-capacity, sustainable physical movement is what's going to take us to our happy promised land of health and capacity. Understand we want to grow this over time. We want to nurture it and grow it responsibly.

So if it's that squat, your goal is to get deeper and deeper over time. It's not about going as deep as I can, and then deeper still, and holding a painful position out of pride or a warped sense of responsibility. Don't override your body's natural wisdom, and just hope that after a while it will feel better.

Instead, squat until your body stops you, or even just a bit before. Stay there, and pay attention to the experience. Notice sensation. Notice tightness, and heat, and tremoring, and ache. Notice balance, and breathing, and numbness, and mood. Respect your current limit. Put all your attention on that edge.

Doing that, you'll get maximum benefit from the exercise. And you'll probably be able to go a bit deeper tomorrow.

Forget about your ego telling you to get all the way to your heels. You want to grow a healthy and capable body like a plant, not build it out of Legos. Don't hurt yourself doing movements designed to heal you.

These are meant to love you and to love your physical parts and pieces as you ask enormous things from them.

6

MOVEMENT

Look, I know I'm an ultra marathoner and I'm excited about running.

I talk about it all the time. I want everybody to enjoy exactly what I enjoy the way I enjoy it, but it doesn't start there.

You're not going to go, "I want to run with you, Josh, so let's run tomorrow." No, we can get together tomorrow, but what we're going to do more than likely is walk - and that's okay.

Start with walking.

I hear so many people downplay their walks:

"Yeah, I know. I'm still just walking."

"I only walked a quarter of a mile."

"I'm not running yet; all I can do is walk right now."

What the fuck you mean? You weigh 150 extra pounds. That's not *just* walking.

That short walk is quite an endeavor, so embrace it. It is the thing that is going to take you out of this condition that you've gotten yourself into. It is the first step.

And walking is very powerful. Do not discount the effect of long walks. Have you ever walked for a solid hour? Have you ever done it in the woods? Have you ever done it over hills?

Have you ever walked for two hours, three hours, all day? Think about our ancestors. Before we had houses and cars and planes and trains and all of that stuff, all we did was walk.

And it just makes good sense to me that walking has been the way our body has recovered for eons. We can't really afford to sit around when lions are chasing us and the rains are moving and the luscious green things to eat aren't here anymore.

Walking is who we are. Walking is very important.

So be gentle as your move forward with this movement. Understand the power of spreading out your body weight over many steps, over many footfalls. Much like the principle behind why a person isn't skewered on a bed of nails. That bed of nails has a bunch of nails in there. If it had half the nails, the person on the bed of nails would be skewered. It's much the same principle in footfalls, the way I've always thought of it, because remember, I started running when I was 380 pounds.

The more footfalls I make, the more steps I take, the less weight each one of them is bearing. The more steps, the less dynamic pounding is happening to my legs and feet.

The way you keep those footfalls voluminous is to take shorter strides. It means keeping your feet under your hips, under your body, under your center of gravity.

Walking with short strides is going to protect you. It's going to help you keep from hurting yourself. There will be times where you will reach beyond your capacity and get burned a little. I think we all have a little Icarus in us. It's okay, but be gentle with yourself. Be patient. You'll achieve your running equivalent of flight in good time.

We don't want to injure ourselves in a way that derails us and sets us back. That was critical to me when I first started to see that running/jogging/walking was starting to get weight off of me. I was so scared that I remember telling myself in my head, "Josh, you're going to hurt a knee, you're going to do something and everybody's going to be like, I told you so fat ass you shouldn't be running."

I was nervous about that, so I stayed very gentle on my body for maybe some dysfunctional reasons. However, the effect was the same. I was able to gently move my big, heavy body through a lot of miles before I ever sustained anything that resembled my first running "injury."

So when I say movement, I'm talking about walking. I'm talking about bipedalism and exploring the forward edge of whatever your capacity is today.

That's where it's at.

Do not discount the power of pumping health into your body with your legs, constantly picking up and pushing against the earth in bipedal locomotion. It's helpful rhythm-wise in your brain and it's helpful fluid exchange-wise, through your quads and your hamstrings.

This is who we are, people. This is who we are.

Just like the birds fly and the fish swim and snakes slither around, and kangaroos hop, we are bipeds. We're not ultra marathoners. We are bipeds. Every one of us from the oldest one to the youngest one that has mastered the art of bipedalism, we all can do it. And that's where the answer is. That's how we're going to get movement. That is the first step.

Walking can be really boring if you're not used to it. It's the same thing again and again.

If you're used to constant distraction, this will take some getting used it. If you have a walking buddy, and you can make conversation, this will be much easier. But if it's just you, and you don't have a screen in front of you, you can easily become bored.

It's very tempting to tune your mind out and say, "Okay, I'm going to distract my mind with an audiobook or a playlist or a podcast," or "I'm going to be on the treadmill watching the game."

There's a lot of research in the field of habit formation about something called bundling, which is to take a habit that you don't like but you want and to attach it to a reward. Like, "I'm only going to watch Netflix when I'm on my stationary bike. I'm only going to watch Game of Thrones when I'm walking on the treadmill.

You're rewarding yourself for doing this unpleasant thing with your body.

The problem with that is that you can injure ourselves slowly, chronically, over time with each step. If you walk for a mile and it feels okay, but at two miles you start feeling a pain in your hip or numbness in your left toes, that's not from the two miles. That's from something you've been doing to injure yourself subtly on every single step and it just tips into your conscious awareness at that point. It didn't "just happen." It's been manifesting "sub-clinically" all along.

It's like an airplane that takes off and it's one 10th of a degree off. At the end of the takeoff runway, you're not going to notice anything. It might just be a foot or three inches off of the center line. But if you're going across the Atlantic, you may end up in Belgium instead of London.

If you're in the habit of distracting yourself when you walk, you won't pay attention to your body until it overshadows than the thing you're using to distract yourself. Once the pain gets louder than the book, the video, the conversation, then it's too late.

I really want to urge you to be mindful of every step, to notice the first bits of discomfort that could lead to pain rather than waiting until it's a screaming bloody mess.

Don't think of it like, "This is the most boring thing." Instead, let each step be a way of loving yourself. This step and this step and this step. You wouldn't be bored during a massage. You'd be like, "This is great. I love this."

Think of each of your movements as massaging yourself, as healing yourself. If you go for a massage and the massage therapist doesn't ask you about the pressure and just digs their elbow into your mid-back until you scream or until something breaks, that's not a good massage.

When you give yourself a massage, you want to pay attention and keep talking to yourself. It's like that analog about dancing to the music only you can hear. You're not going to be able to do it every single second of every walk, but to the extent that you can, keep checking in.

Pay attention to how each step feels. That way you can make on-the-fly micro-corrections without even having to think about them. You don't have to be an expert in kinetics, in posture and movement. Just being an expert in your own internal compass of this feels good, that feels better, this feels worse.

Love yourself with each step. Take care of yourself on each footfall.

7

RECOVERY

Once we start moving on purpose, with purpose, we often complain about these little nagging pains that happen to us.

I remember complaining a lot about hangovers too, and I still did them.

It's really funny because alcohol feels good right at first and then you feel really crappy after, but running feels really crappy right at first, but it feels really good after, all day long. I think of running sort of like drinking in reverse. And I think that's a very refreshing take on it, because it leads me to think about how many times I have spent the morning after a long night of drinking nursing myself into recovery.

Once you start moving longer and farther, and with more intensity, you'll also wake up sore and aching a bit. Something might be hurting that wasn't hurting yesterday.

A movement hangover, if you will. But now, instead of a handful of Tylenol or I holla the doc, I grab the foam roller or I go get a massage or I sit in a sauna and self-massage. I do something to manipulate my soft tissues and it gets some fluid exchange.

That's how we heal; with fresh blood. Look on YouTube for good ways to foam roll your glutes and IT band and your hamstrings and your quads. Play around with it, find your own little protocol that you create and tweak until it works for you.

Foam rolling is key, because it's an efficient means of getting fresh blood to all of that tissue to help it heal properly, to help it have oxygen and nutrients and all of the stuff that is in that beautiful red liquid.

But we also want to make sure that that red liquid, our life's blood, is rich with healing power because of our food. We want to make sure that after we do something that makes us super sore and tight and tired, that we fuel our body in a very anti-inflammatory way. Google it, Google anti-inflammatory foods and hit the Images tab.

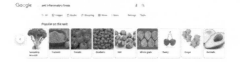

That's how I did it. I would always make sure I was staying in an anti-inflammatory category. It's very important to keep your blood right, right? It's cool to get massages and all, but we want to make sure we get the right shit in that blood. It feels good.

For a lot more information about the best foods for athletic performance and recovery, as well as losing weight and even reversing chronic disease, check out our first book, *Sick to Fit*. We've got a whole Menu chapter in there.

The way we keep that blood right is we make sure that we are as clean as possible. You might misbehave from time to time and have little slip-ups and have little packaged things from here, there, or whatever. Don't sweat it – instead, focus on your overall dietary pattern.

Especially in those moments when you're really hurting and you know you've really put your body through a lot, that's when it's most important to get your food right.

It's not the way we're taught to think about eating. Most runners, even experienced ones, think about a long run as an opportunity to eat whatever they want because they've just "earned" it. If you have a calories in, calories out, mindset that leads to you binge on your old favorites as a reward for burning calories through movement, you'll miss a huge opportunity to take care of your body.

After a workout, eat clean.

That's when your body needs optimal nutrition the most, when it's dealing with all sorts of toxins that it just mobilized from the body fat it consumed as fuel. That's when it needs to create new red blood cells. That's when it needs to break apart old tissue, and synthesize new tissue.

Think of every workout as a tiny remodeling project for your body. You get to decide if your new building materials will be high quality, or the cheapest shit you can find. Whatever you decide, that's the house you're going to live with, and in, from now on. You can't move out. You can only take the best care you can of what you've got.

It's so important to make sure you have enough greens in our diet, and water to help flush toxins. Just water, clean water, nothing extra in it for the liver to filter. No hacks, no recovery drinks, no special teas, no special recovery blend. Chocolate milk is not necessary.

Recovery is a very important part of growth. Some of the most powerful runners I know often share the quote that recovery is where strength is built.

In *Peak Performance*, Brad Stulberg and Steve Magness introduced their "Growth Equation":

Stress + Rest = Growth

We understand from the last chapter the power of strength. Well, the most powerful thing you can do for your strength is proper recovery. So give yourself plenty of time to recover, especially when you're still heavy.

I run six days a week now, but back when I was first starting, I was nervous to run more than two or three days a week. I had a rule where I didn't run two days in a row, ever.

You might be there on your continuum. You might need to do even less than that. Whatever it is, wherever you are, build the off day or off days into your training schedule.

Depending on where you are, give yourself the time necessary to let your body do the miracles inside that it takes to recover.

And in this process, if you're doing it right, you should be tired. You should want to go to bed early. Don't fight it. DVR that favorite show of yours or better yet, just skip it.

Turn it into a running fan .

But seriously, if you get up early and you attend to your movement and you're doing things on purpose to make yourself stronger and looser, and you're going to early morning yoga classes, and you go and have a full day at work, and then you get home and eat supper - man, you should be getting tired. You should be ready to go to bed.

And we need to be aiming to go to bed as soon as we can when we get home. Those rhythms of going to sleep soon after dark and waking up right before daylight or right at daylight are crucial to our evolution. It's what authentic humans did before we became reliant on climate-controlled shelters and electric lights.

Don't fight being tired. Embrace it, search it out. Try to *make* yourself tired with your movement. That's a wonderful tool to get yourself prepped for bed.

You start prepping for that bedtime as soon as you hit your feet on the ground in the morning, and you get no better recovery than the recovery you get in REM sleep. Look it up.

If you want to supercharge your recovery protocol, we need more sleep. Embrace the awkwardness of that. I know it feels wrong, but you need to figure out a way to get to bed earlier. It's just that simple. It'll pay dividends in your life.

Game of Thrones isn't that important. Like we would say on the bayou, it's time to make the dough. So close the iPad, close the laptop, forget about CNN for right now, let those eyes be heavy.

Time to create that practice of getting to bed at an uncomfortably early time so you can start waking up at this new uncomfortably early time. That's your "life hack" that will allow you to get your movement in and build your strength and be the thing that you say you want to be, to have the capacity that's going to benefit those around you. It's all built in recovery.

FUCK YOU

If you're like me and my brother and many other people that I know in my life, people who have been heavy most of their lives, you've been picked on.

Hell, everybody's probably been picked on and made fun of at one time or another in their life. But I suspect that fat people get a disproportionate amount of teasing and being marginalized and made fun of.

You know exactly what I'm talking about. The cruel remarks. The coded words. The subtle put-downs. The embarrassed looks.

We get conditioned as kids. We hear it so much from adults and from principals and from parents and from grandparents and aunts, and kids on the school yard, and we hear it over and over again, and we think we're ignoring it or you think we've become numb to it. But what we wind up doing, I find, is we become complicit.

You wind up carrying the ball for those assholes when they're not around. They're not around to make fun of you, they're not around to degrade you.

So what do you do when you stand in front of the mirror? "You fat piece of shit. Look at you." I know I did it. That voice is powerful. It holds you back, it holds you down. It tells you you can't, it tells you won't. It tells you, "You don't have the gumption; you haven't got the moxie, son."

And that voice isn't you. You think it is, because it's in your head and sometimes comes out of your mouth. But it's not.

It's not you; you have been tricked into being complicit. You have been tricked just through sheer volume of repetitions, to participate in this violent rhetoric against yourself.

And when you're alone and you're working really hard and you're scared and you're hurting, and you feel like you can't, just think about it.

Think about that voice that's saying, " I told you that you wouldn't. I told you that you couldn't."

Just think about all of the people that went into that single voice in your head. Because that voice is really just an amalgamation of all the people who have fucking fucked with you all your life. They've embedded this voice inside you.

And at every decision point, in every moment where you're going to do something different, whether it's how you move or how you eat or how you think, you have the opportunity to scream at the top of your lungs to everyone who doubted you, "Fuck you. You think I won't, you think I can't. Hide and watch this, player."

That is a very powerful dynamic.

Once you stick to loving yourself and moving yourself forward through the failures and creating a progress that creates the outcomes you dream of, that makes you fitter and makes you lighter, that makes you stronger, makes you healthier, then you become a beacon.

Then you become a person that people seek: "How'd you do it?"

And some of those people who are now asking for your advice are the very people who contributed to that voice, that old voice that used to hold you down. They are the ones that told you that you couldn't. They are the ones that make you feel less than. They are the ones who shamed you for being fat and for being a glutton and a lazy-ass.

And now you have the opportunity to watch them squirm as they try their best not to ask you for advice because the tables have turned. That is a beautiful moment, and I wish that for you more than you can imagine.

I'm in love with that idea more than I'm in love with the fact that we got to name a chapter, "Fuck You."

This is what I desperately want you to understand: You are your answer.

You are how you are going to get out of this.

You are the fucking hero of this story and to any voice that says otherwise: "Fuck You."

When you're alone and that voice creeps in and now you're empowered with the understanding that the voice is not you, the voice is a collection of all those assholes in your life, you get to respond to that voice with a great big Fuck You.

But your true Fuck You isn't said in words.

Your deepest Fuck You is expressed by your decision to take that next step in your walk and not quit just because you're bored or tired.

Your most authentic Fuck You is when you grab a bag of broccoli and some mustard for dipping sauce instead of chicken nuggets and sweet and sour sauce like the assholes think you're going to do, like that voice in your head that's taking up for those clowns thinks you're going to do.

Each time you make one of those decisions, each time you step the other way *on* purpose *with* purpose; each time you do that, you are loving yourself with a very solid, loud and clear Fuck You to everything and everyone that tried to stop you.

We'll get caught in moments where that voice tells us you're not doing it right, you may as well just quit. That voice says, you'll never be X. You'll never be fit. You'll never be an athlete. You'll never be good looking. Whatever.

It will point to the less-than-perfect result of the thing you just tried, whether it's a pot of rice you cooked for the first time and totally burned it, or your first attempt to walk around the block for the first time and you had to get a ride home.

That voice will say, in a totally predictable fashion, "This isn't for you. You are never going to get it figured out."

My wife and I have what we call our "fuck it bucket." It's one of our most valuable imaginary possessions. It's where we toss all our failures, our mistakes, our missteps, our accidents. All our useful, valuable, necessary-to-success fuckups.

Get yourself a fuck it bucket. Toss that shit in there. Appreciate them for what they were, for what they taught you about doing better next time. And at the end of the day, throw them out, say "fuck it," and move on.

Move on. Get back up. Dust yourself off and return to the journey. That moment is the loudest Fuck You of all to the voice that puts you down and predicts failure.

Turn each Fuck It into a Fuck You: "You think I'm going to keep failing because I just made a mistake? You think that's all I got? I can and will take steps to move out of that. I can and will take steps to move forward from this."

You have the power to decide that this time is different from the times in the past where you gave up when things got hard or didn't go your way.

And as you take those steps, literal or figurative, each footfall is a Fuck... You... Fuck... You... Fuck... You...

Just like I want to spread out my footfalls over a run when I'm big and heavy, I also want to spread out those decisions. I want to make sure that I have a bunch of them, to take the pressure of any single one.

If I have a thousand tests in a semester, I have a thousand chances to bring up my average. So look at every single tiny little thing in your life as a win or a loss.

It's not just three meals a day, it's every single decision that you make. How close to the grocery store door did I park? What did I grab out of the vending machine at work? Did I stick to my bedtime, or stay up scrolling Instagram?

Make sure you have so many chances to make good decisions that you can't help stack up some Ws each day, wins that represent your intention to create a better outcome for yourself.

Every single tiny decision matters. Each one is a potential Fuck You to the nasty, defeated, bully voice inside you.

Did I even touch the vending machine today? Every single tiny decision.

Did I drink water instead of grabbing a diet Coke? Every single tiny decision.

You don't have to manufacture these decision points; they already exist, and they are legion. Instead, your job is to be aware of them, to be present for them, to understand the opportunity they represent.

And to bring your Fuck You energy into as many of those decision points as you can, so we can chalk up as many Ws as possible.

You want to build momentum with all these small wins to help prove to yourself that you aren't just faking the funk. That your Fuck You isn't just words.

This is deep. This is real. Live it out loud with your body. The words themselves are almost moot.

Actions, as we know, speak louder than words. Your actions that override your old default behaviors scream loudly. They are the means by which you build a new relationship with yourself. They are how you become your own leader.

Harnessing the power of the action-based Fuck You has been very powerful for me in my life. It may sound dysfunctional and angry and violent, but goddammit, it is useful.

And we don't stop there...

9

LOVE ME

I know that last chapter sounded very angry and violent and probably unprofessional as hell.

I don't really care. It comes from my heart.

The heart is maybe a funny place for a Fuck You to originate. But would you agree that there's a certain anger that you feel when you witness someone you love being hurt?

Imagine someone hitting your mom. Really take a moment to picture it. Does it make you angry?

Here's the thing: the anger associated with somebody hitting your mom is directly proportional to the love you have for her.

The more we love someone, the more rage we can experience when we witness a boundary violation of that person.

You're also a person.

And all that name-calling and abuse and "good-natured" kidding at your expense was nothing if not a never-ending gauntlet of boundary violations.

I think it's healthy to experience that kind of anger on your own behalf. Finally.

It's love-borne anger.

You finally are seeing the abuse you suffered, in a way maybe you never realized before now. And the depth of your Fuck You at the thought of that abuse is equal to the height of the love you can feel for yourself.

The outward Fuck You is simply a reflection of the inward Love Me.

That Love Me was the engine of my transformation. For the first time ever in my life, I could say "I love me, truly, Joshua."

That love led me to the moxie and the gumption necessary to put all of those Fuck You's out of the ether.

How to Love Me

I make no bones about the fact that a key factor in my journey was seeing a therapist, about getting help. Because early on, and even after I had already lost a lot of weight, I still had a very bad dysfunctional relationship with not only people in my family, but with myself.

I went to a therapist about it and we talked and we discussed and we discovered that I often felt unsafe in my childhood. He had me do an exercise in his office where he had me imagine the 5-year-old boy that I used to be. I pictured myself as a scared little boy worried that I just spilled the milk, and about how angry daddy is, and what's that whipping going to be like.

He had me sit that little boy down in a chair next to me and look at him in the eyes and tell him, "I love you. And I got your fucking back.

nd we can finally be happy. You don't have to worry. I'm a grown ass man and I can take care of you."

If you can see yourself as that helpless little boy or girl, worried sick, confused about life, not sure how to take these things that are happening, and you can have his or her tiny little back, then you understand the power of the Fuck You to anyone and anything that would threaten or hurt that child.

The volume of that Fuck You, the gutturalness of that Fuck You, is proof of how much I Love Me.

Not Just Words

I could go around saying Fuck You to everybody. (I kind of do anyway.)

But I could go around just saying the words, Fuck You. That's not the point here. The genuine Fuck You was born out of loving me.

It's like digging a hole. I got the shovel and I'm digging a hole and each scoop is a Fuck You. When I take that shovel load of dirt and I throw it up on the side of the hole, that's all love. Those two things are very much connected. I can do the rhetoric, I can say the words, but they're empty without the love. Fuck You doesn't work unless it's powered by Love Me.

The Healthy at Any Size movement tells is that moderation and body positivity are the same thing as self-love.

As we saw in Chapter 3, these philosophies can tease you into accepting the fact that you're unhealthy and overweight and unhappy, and have you do some sort of rhetorical trick to convince others through words that you have a positive image of this body you hate.

You can say, "I love me, I love me, I love me," but until you stick a foot in the sand and actually do the first thing, put action where your words are, it's all just a game. It's just a facade.

Action doesn't have to be a race, where you're running at 100% intensity. Action doesn't have to be a marathon, where you push yourself to keep going past all prior limits.

That action, that first proof of self-love can happen at the gas station you're about to stop at, or at the cafe you're about to go to lunch to, or at the running track you're about to drive away from because you're just too tired.

That first proof of love is in what you do. My wife keeps a sign on her office wall that says, "Actions speak louder than words, so sit down and shut up."

Let's amend it to, "Actions speak louder than words, so stand up and scream, 'I love me' with our actions."

I have truly tried to do that in my life. Not just say that I love Joshua for the first time, because I did that for a while, but to truly prove I love him by how I behave.

To prove my love for Joshua by how I nurture my body.

By how I'm not willing to wreck myself to look cool to others or to be impressive to others.

That's what makes talking about all of this so hard. The words are such a tiny part. They're such a tiny part.

The big part is the movement, the doing, the action; regardless of how tiny you may think it is. Regardless of how minuscule that voice in your head wants to make it, that first little action is your first Love Me. Keep screaming it every day - it'll change your life.

Gratitudes

I'm standing here in my very good friend Howard's house after an amazing weekend. We just wrapped up our first Sick to Fit retreat, having spent some time with a dozen people struggling with some of these things that I wrote about here.

I feel on top of the world, I feel amazing about how things are lining up for me in my mind and how I'm been able to convey messages to people in packages that seem to be digestible and implementable in your lives.

It's been an awakening for me. It's my rebirth as a whole new human being. I understand the heaviness and the workload ahead for you. I know what I can feel like when you're trying to lose so much weight and change your life in a big way when you have all the pressures of family and culture and habit and identity. I get it.

This book is very important for me. This book is a way for me to speak in real time with no preparation. I didn't write this out and think about it. Instead, I just recorded it as sort of stream of consciousness, and Howie edited the manuscript from there.

If you want to hear the unfiltered rants that were the origin of this book, you can find the audio version on Audible.

This book is a way to give myself some therapy, a way to get some things out of me that I haven't really shared a whole lot about.

It's a way to be vulnerable for myself, but at the same time try to stand up and have a backbone and do something courageous for people that I know are looking my way for some answers.

I'm trying to give you all the answers I can give you. I'm trying to share every nugget of every nuance, little piece of my story that I think might help along the way.

I want to take a minute to thank Howie for his help with this book, and with everything that we're doing together. He knows where people's blind spots are, so he knows what he wants me to help with.

It's a very wonderful thing to see in my life to not only have this experience to share, but to also have a partner with not only the ability to help me share it, but what seems like a burning desire to help me share it.

I want to thank you, the reader, for being a part of what Howie and I are trying to build going forward. I want this book to just be another little package filled with nuggets for you to use as you take your next step forward in this journey. I hope it's been useful to you and above all, I hope I can move the needle just a hair on how you think about yourself.

If you're like I was, you haven't thought about the miracles going on in your body. You haven't thought about how amazing you are.

We're too busy thinking about bad things to realize that we literally are miracles.

Even though I've been doing all of this rough stuff to my body, these beautiful chemical things have been happening in body to keep me alive and relatively healthy. My endocrine system is a fucking miracle. I have no idea how it does it.

These beautiful things, these organs have been working in a certain way to keep me healthy. Holy shit, I am a miracle.

I'm not a fat ass; I'm not lazy. That's just a toxic story that got put into my head like a virus.

I have participated in some behaviors that got me into a bad spot, but goddammit. Here I am with my eyes wide open and I'm looking for answers.

I'm not wishing anymore. I'm doing. And for that I say thank you.

It feels good to have people headed with me in the direction of better, more authentic, happier, healthier. And regardless of where you are on a continuum (you may have just been able to start standing up yesterday), this is going to sound weird, but I truly love you.

I love you because I get it and I know what you're going through and I know you can make it out. So I'll hold that spot for you.

I'll love you until you can heed my words here and do the things that prove you love you too.

If it's helpful, follow me. Come along with me on my journey. Stay in touch with me on social media. Message me.

I want to be your friend. I want to help you out.

And I hope this book helps. I really do.

Peace. I love you.

Made in United States
Orlando, FL
16 March 2023